Nurse Ted
A Children's Guide to Brain Tumours

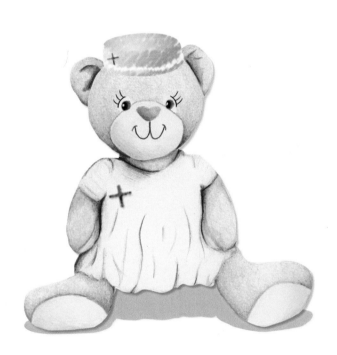

Ffion Jones ● Kerry Foster-Mitchell

With thanks to the Royal Surrey County Hospital,

Dr Shaffer, and the Neuro-Oncology Team for all their support.

www.nurseted.com

First Published 2015 by Belrose Books. Copyright © 2015 Nurse Ted Ltd in accordance

with the Copyright, Designs and Patents Act, 1988.

"Nurse Ted" story text and illustrations by Ffion Jones. www.ffijones.com

The moral rights of Ffion Jones to be identified as author/ illustrator of the "Nurse Ted"

story have been asserted.

Photographs, Glossary, Parent's/Carer's Guide, Questions and Answers page (text), Side

Effects page by Kerry Foster-Mitchell. Her moral rights have been asserted.

ISBN 978-0-9931579-0-5

Disclaimer: The "Nurse Ted" story is a work of fiction. Names, characters, places, and incidents are either products

of the author's imagination or used fictitiously. "Nurse Ted" has been written for informational purposes only and

should not be used for diagnosing or treating a health problem. If the reader thinks they may have a health problem,

they should consult with their healthcare provider. The information given in the book is considered to be current and

relevant in the Royal Surrey County Hospital at the time of printing and has been obtained from reliable sources.

However, neither the publisher nor its authors guarantee accuracy or completeness of any information published herein

and neither the publisher nor its authors shall be responsible to any party for any errors, omissions, or claims for damage

with regard to the accuracy or sufficiency of the information contained in the book. Neither the publisher nor its authors

are responsible for any consequences that may occur if readers follow the suggestions in the book. The book may not be

suitable for everyone who is affected by a brain tumour.

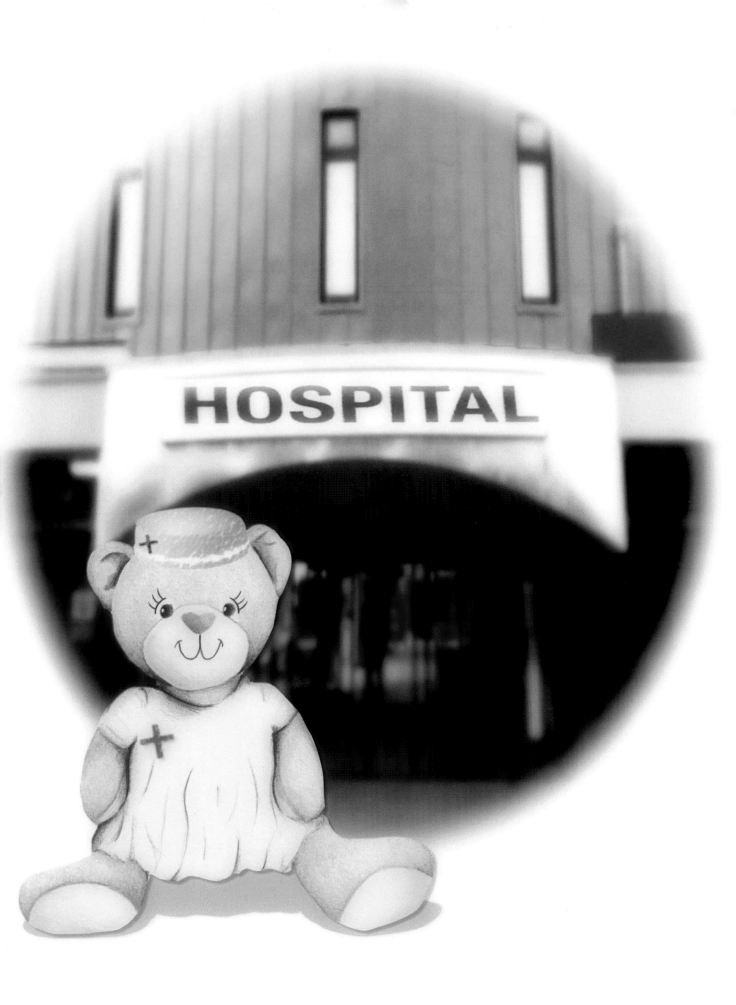

I'm Nurse Ted and I work here at the hospital.

I like working here because **I** like helping people to get better when they're sick.

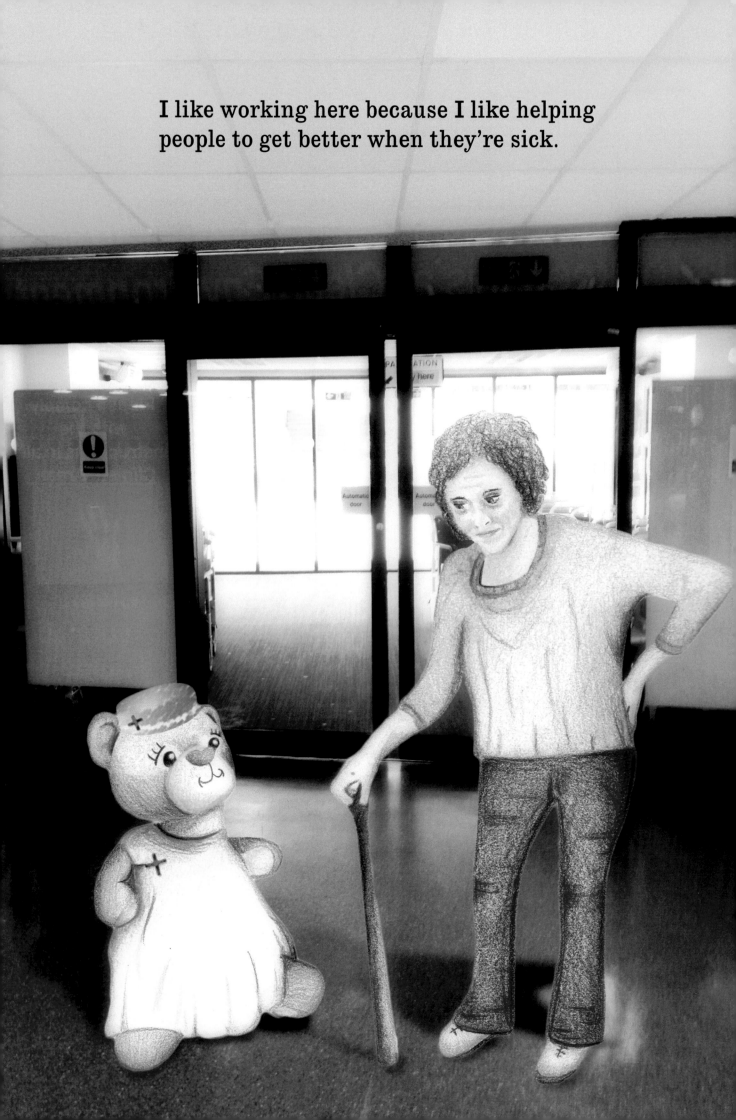

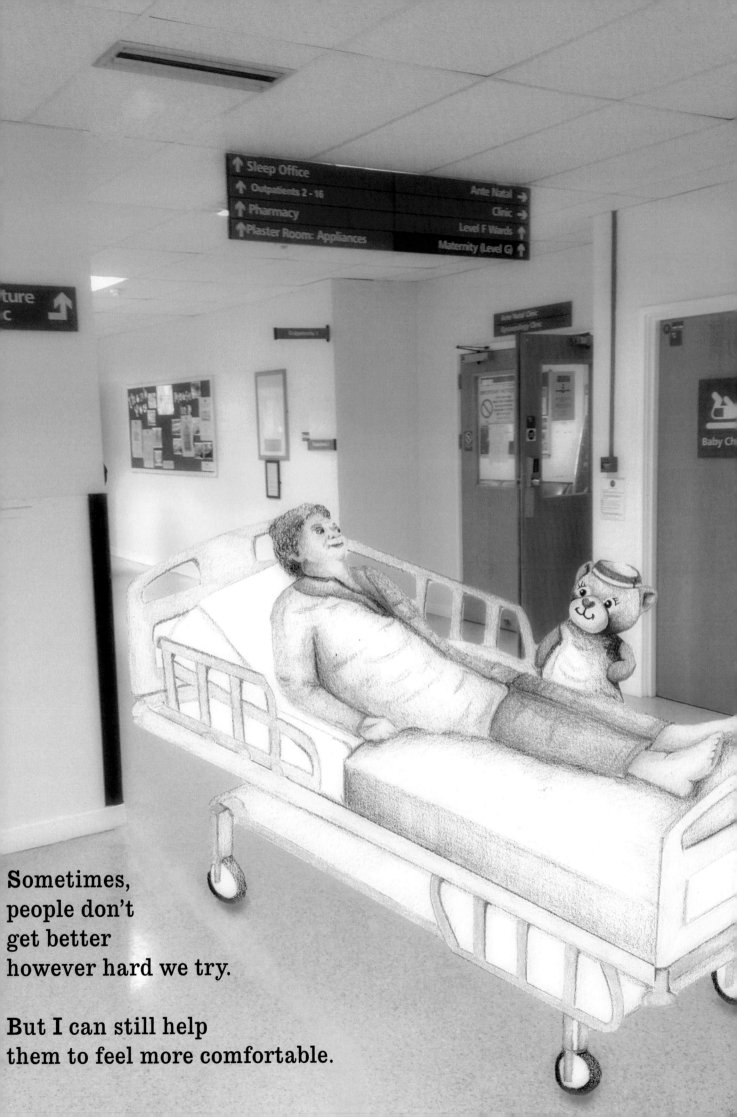

Sometimes, people don't get better however hard we try.

But I can still help them to feel more comfortable.

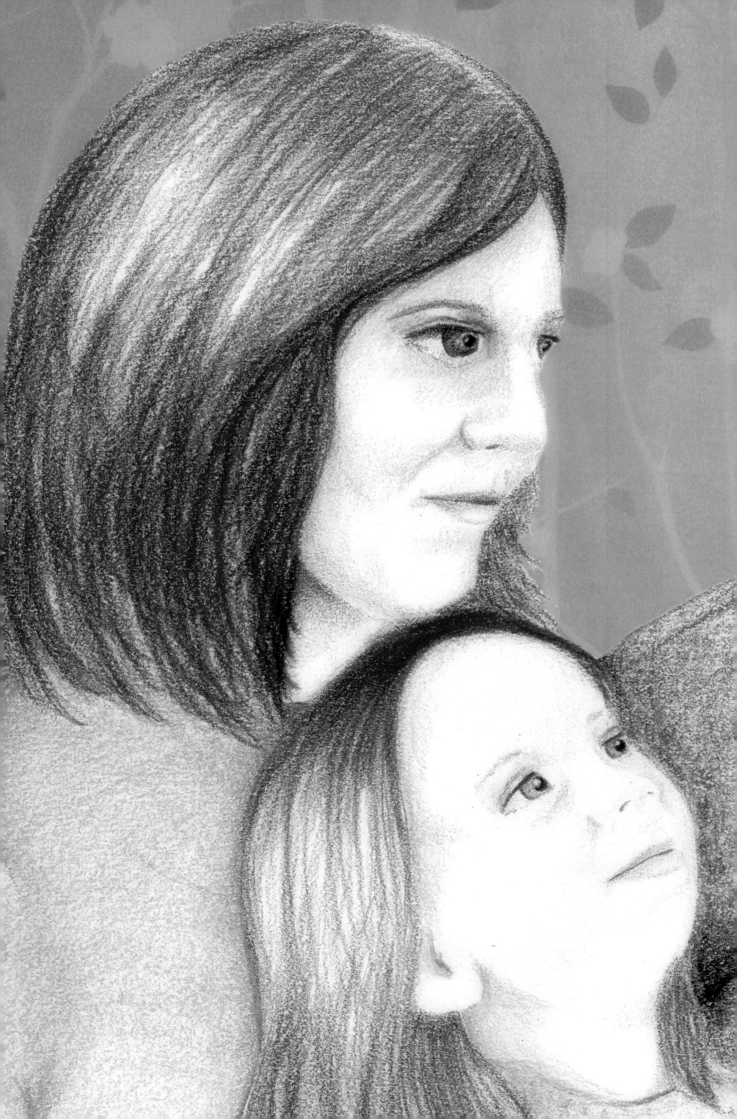

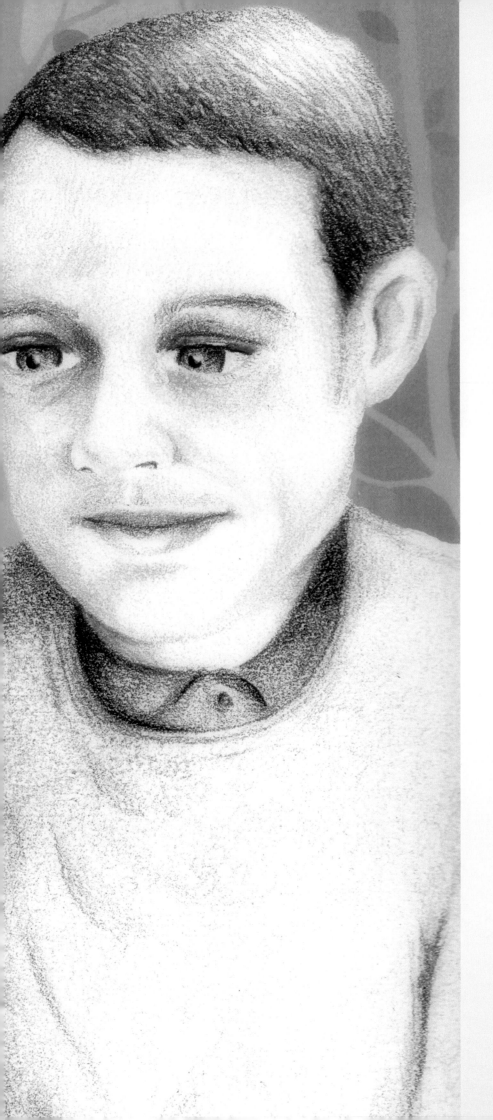

Lilly's dad started
to visit us at the
hospital when his
head started
to hurt.

He lives with Lilly
and her mum who
always try to make
him smile.

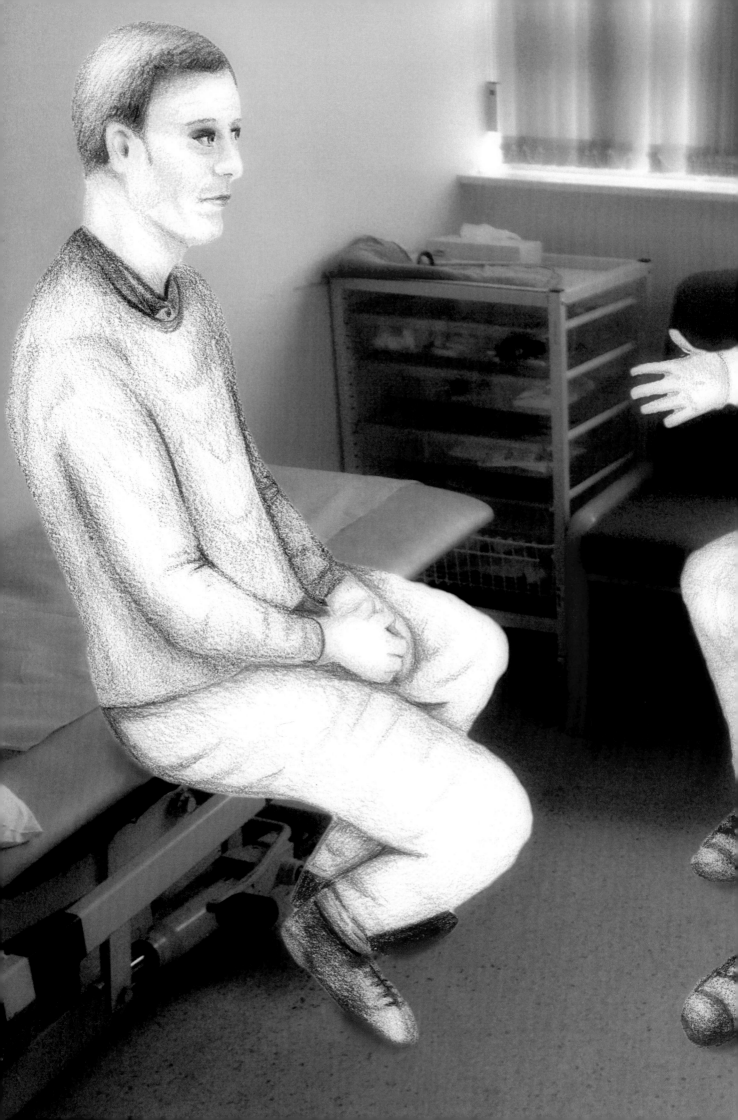

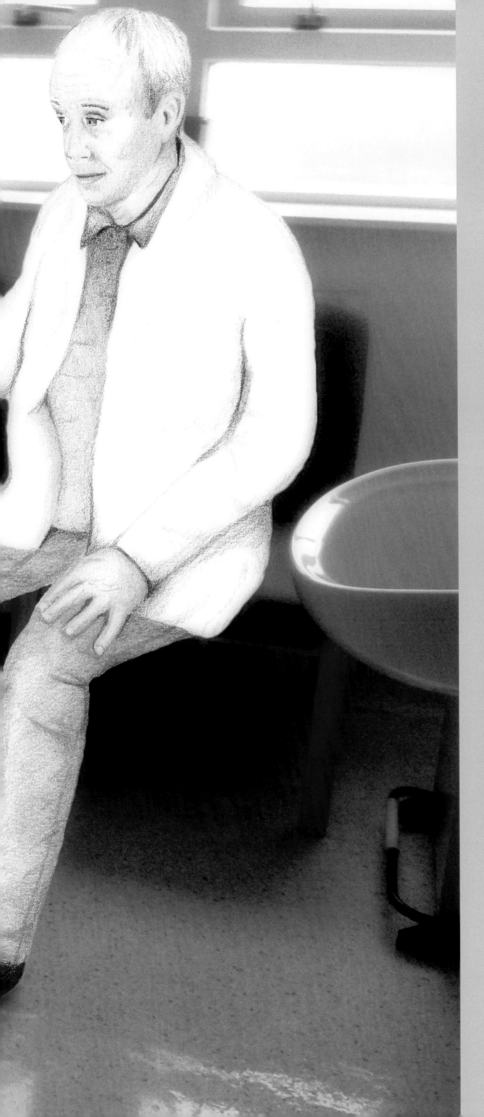

He went to see his doctor as soon as he started having headaches and feeling sick.

He also had a seizure, when his body shook all over. This made Lilly and her mum feel worried and scared.

The doctor said his body wasn't working properly and sent him to see us at the hospital.

We have special tests and machines to help us find out what's wrong with people's bodies.

Lilly's dad had one of these tests called a brain scan. He had to stay very still when he was having the scan.

It took pictures, like a camera, of the inside of his head.

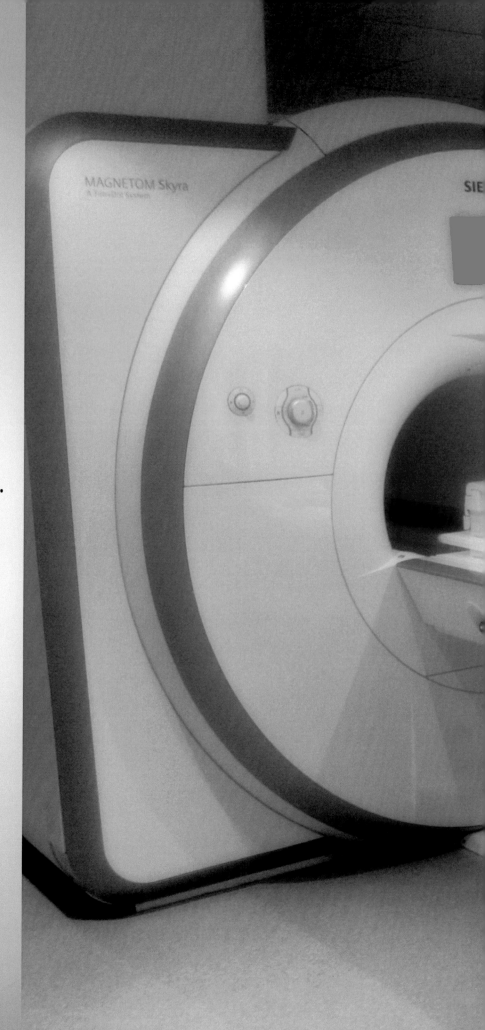

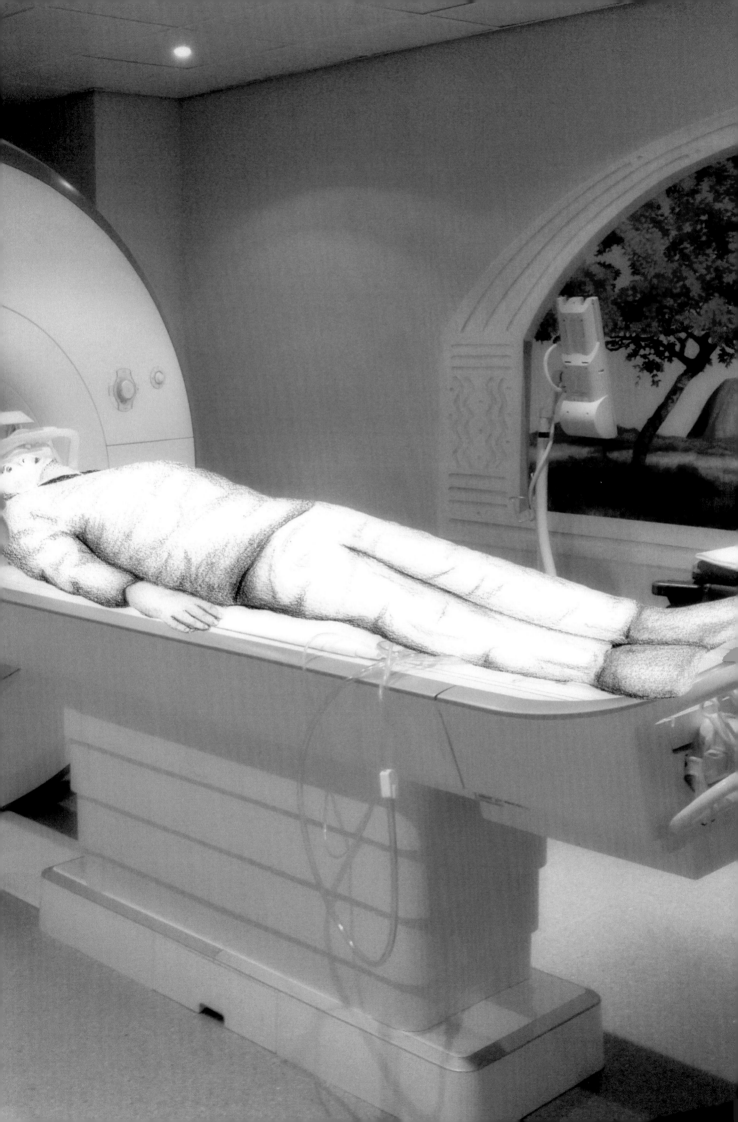

We looked at the pictures and saw a lump that was causing his sickness.

The lump is called a brain tumour.

Some brain tumours are not cancer.

But Lilly's dad's tumour was a type of cancer in his head.

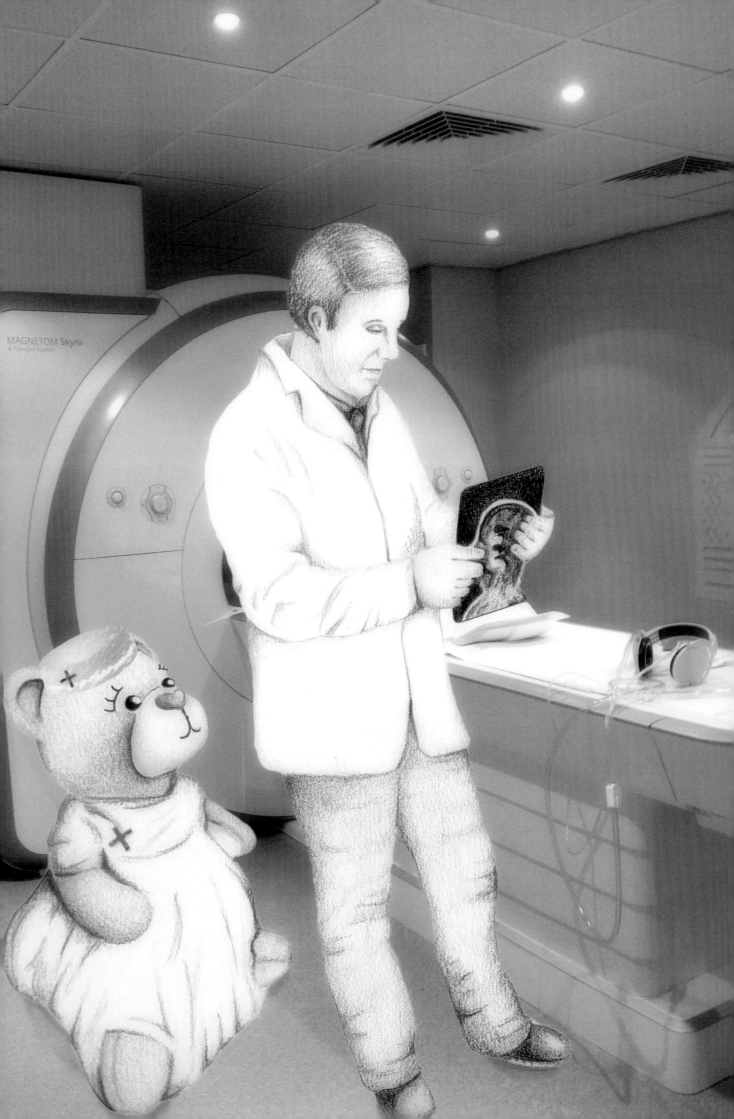

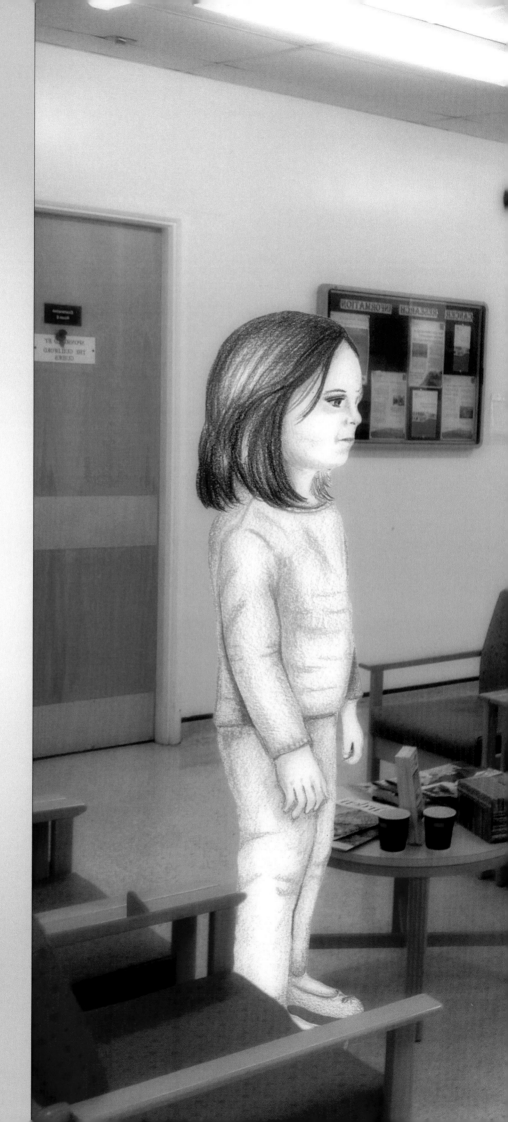

"What's cancer?"
Lilly asked
because she felt
a little scared.

"You'll feel less
scared," I told her,
"once I've
explained it all
to you."

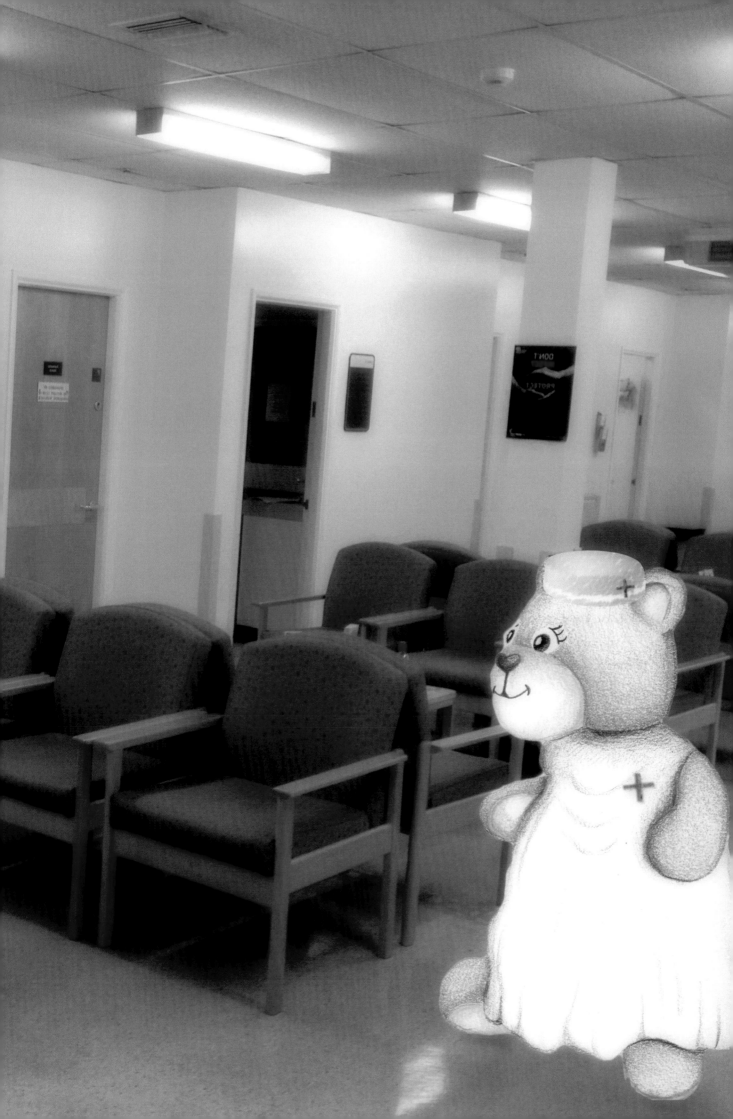

"Everyone is made up of trillions of tiny things called cells," I said, "which all have a special job to do to make your body work properly. But sometimes cells can get sick, just like we can."

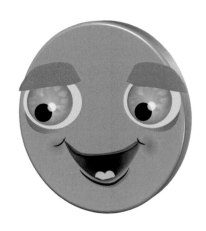

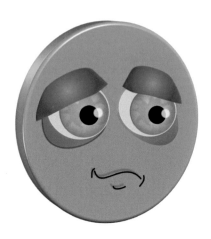

"We don't always know why and it's nobody's fault; sometimes cells just grow when they shouldn't."

"The sick cells can join up to make a lump, called a tumour. The tumour can stop the healthy cells from working properly, making the person feel sick."

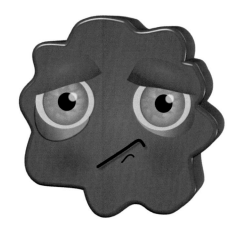

"Now we have found your daddy's tumour," I explained,
"we can try to help him in three different ways:
an operation, radiotherapy, and chemotherapy.
Sometimes, the sick cells can be quite strong so we try
to get rid of them in more than one way."

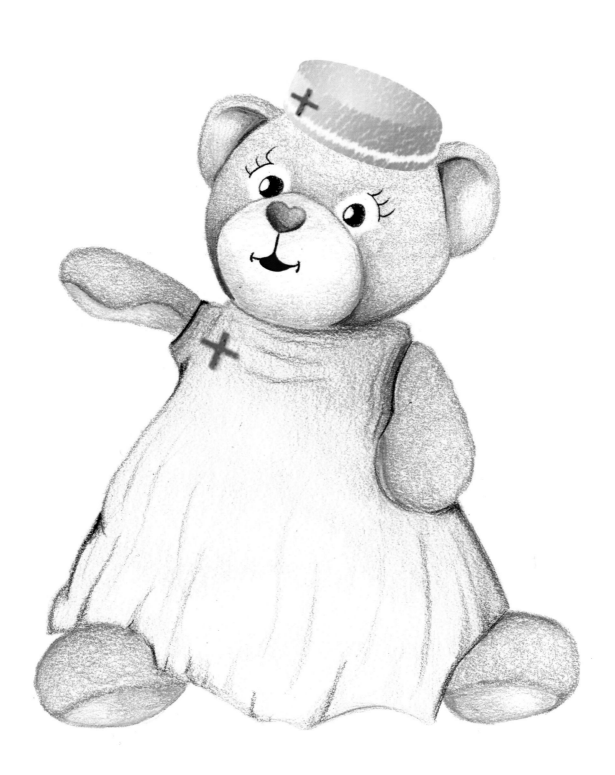

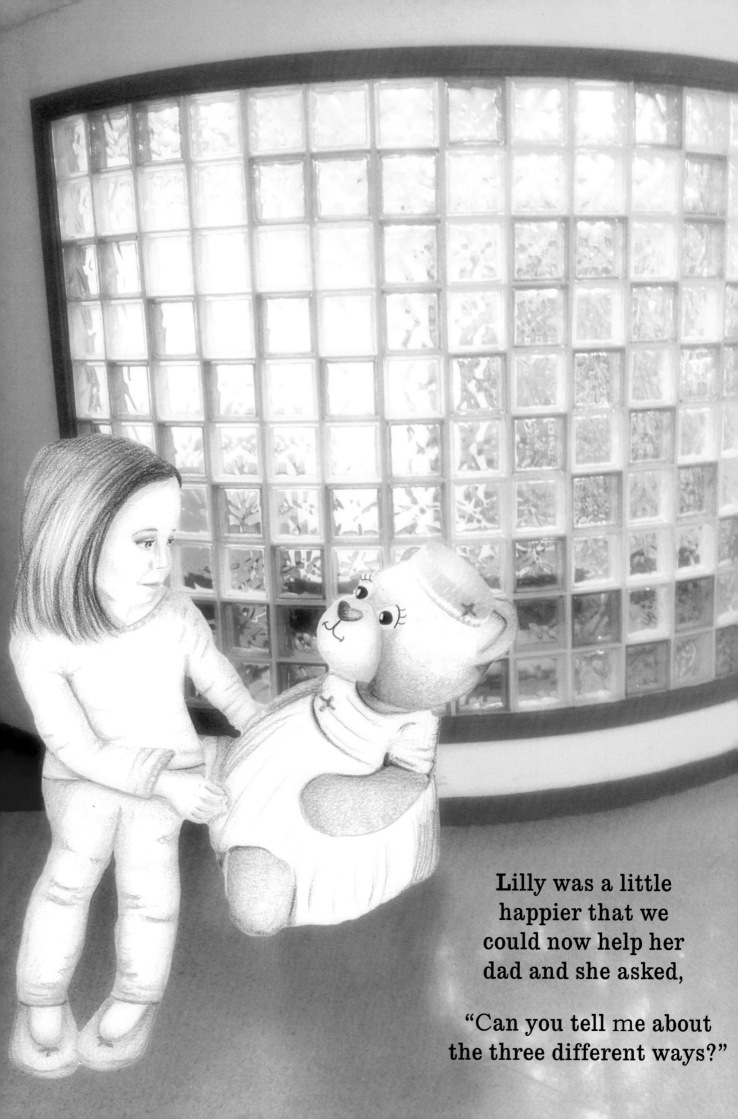

Lilly was a little happier that we could now help her dad and she asked,

"Can you tell me about the three different ways?"

"It's good to ask questions," I said, "because talking through what may happen can make you feel less scared."

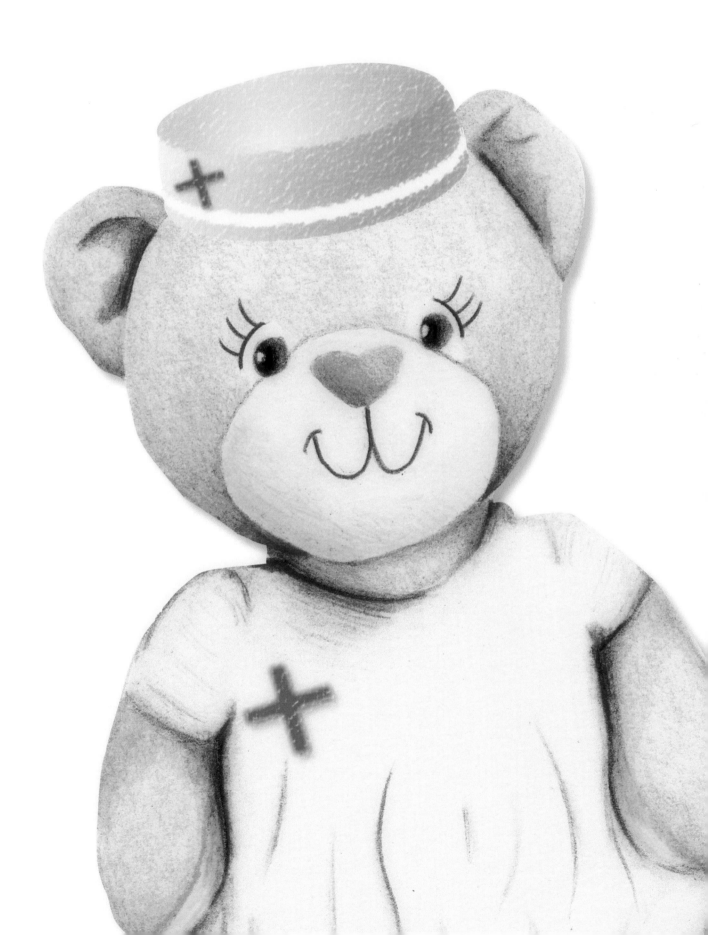

"First of all," I explained, "your daddy will have an operation to try to take some of the tumour out."

"He will have to stay in hospital for a while, but when he is here we will help him to feel better."

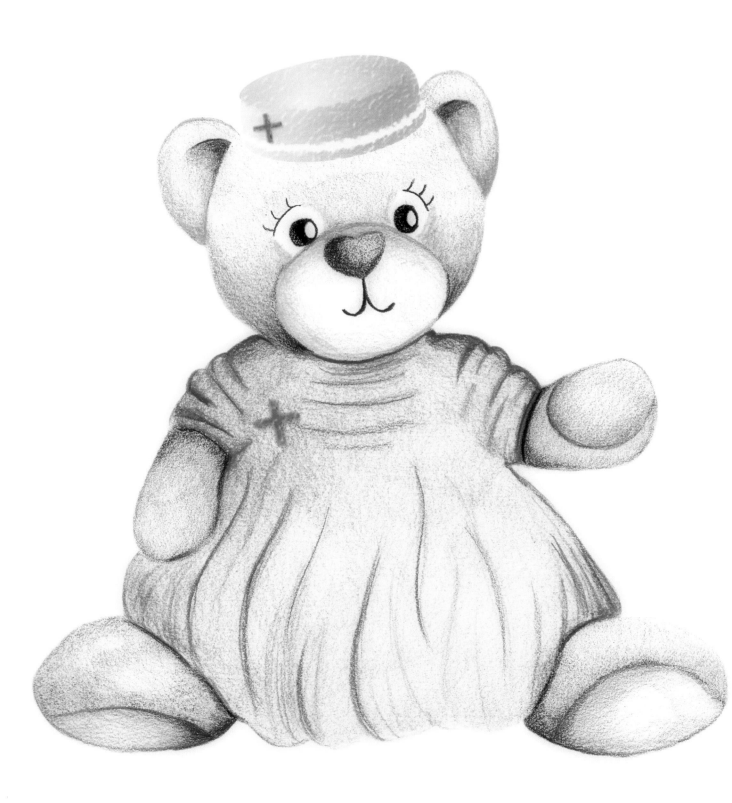

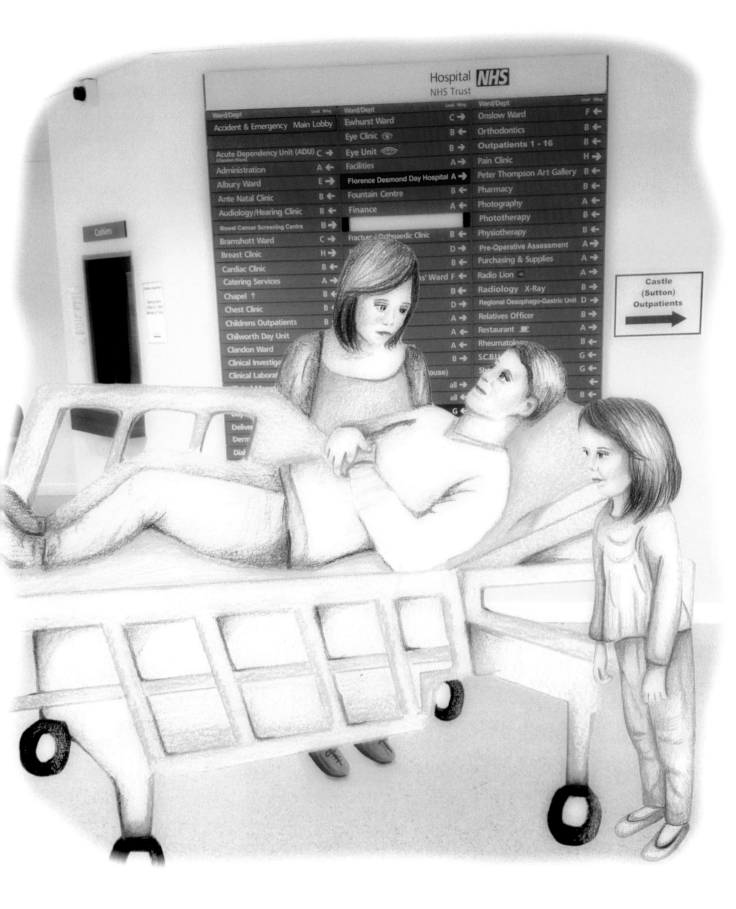

Lilly was sad the first time her dad stayed with us at the hospital because she missed him and their cuddles.

But she knew that he was in the best place.

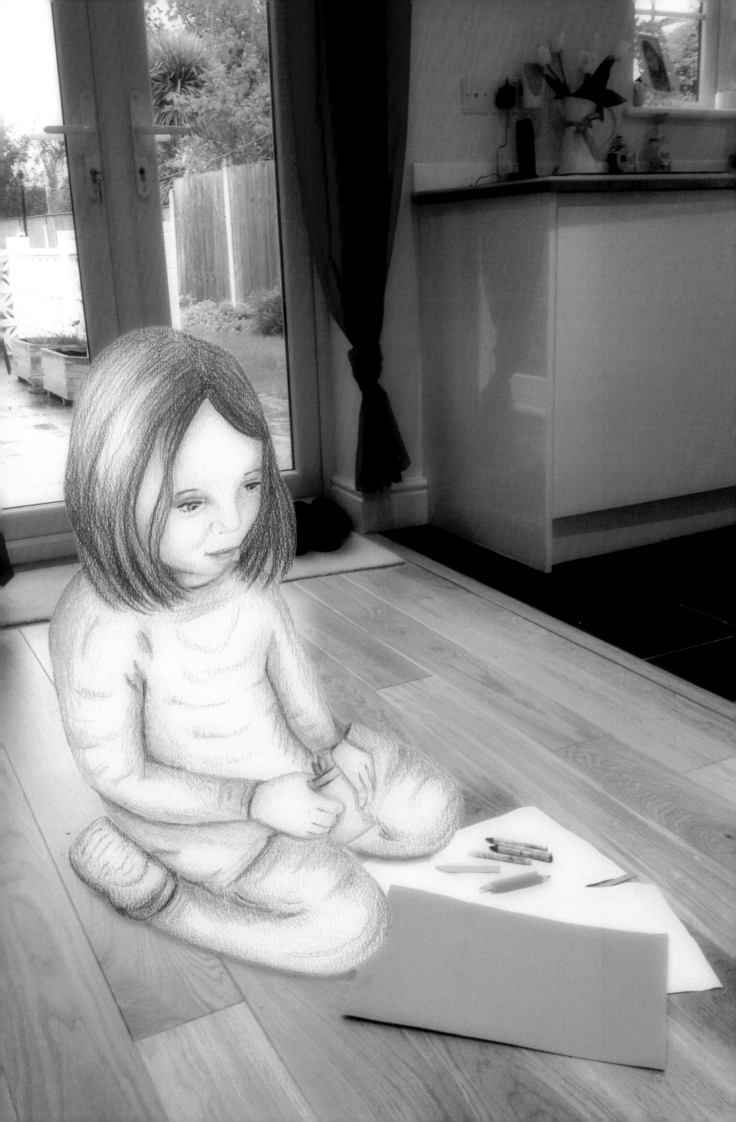

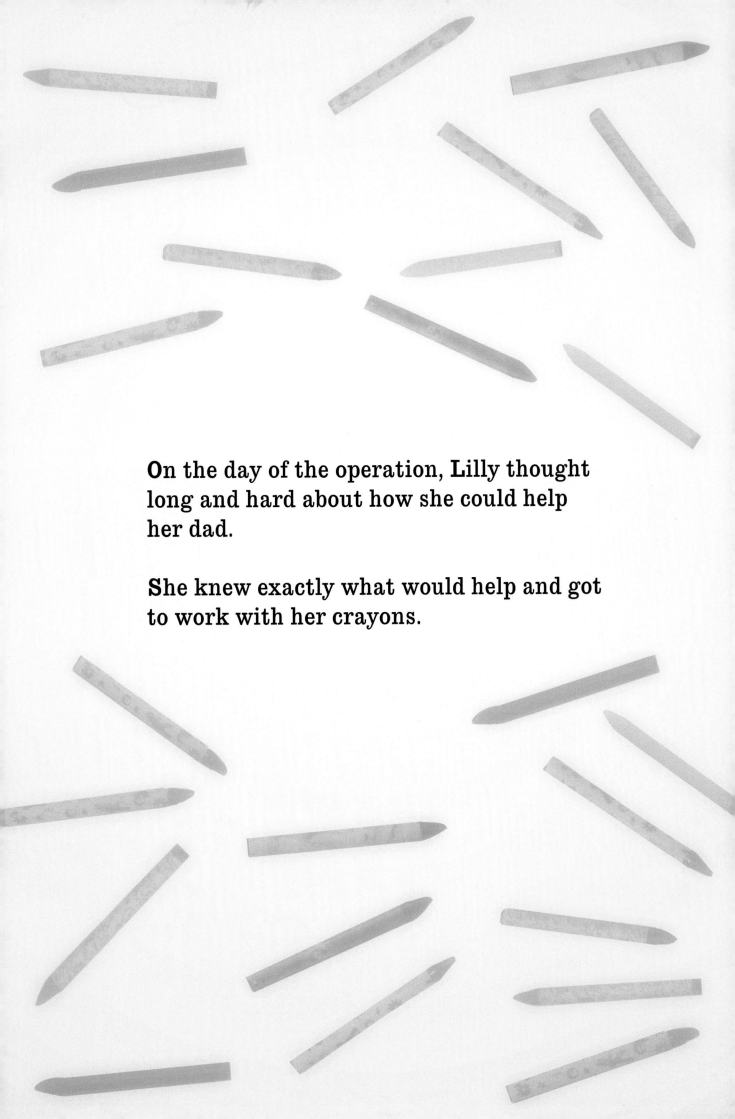

On the day of the operation, Lilly thought long and hard about how she could help her dad.

She knew exactly what would help and got to work with her crayons.

When he woke up from the operation, Lilly's dad
was tired and a little sore.

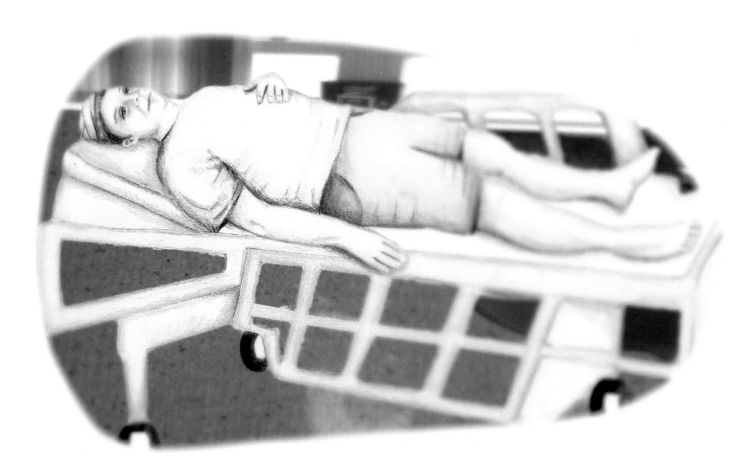

He stayed in a special ward called "Intensive Care"
so that the nurses could keep an eye on him and give him
medicine to make him feel better.

Soon he was back on another ward and Lilly came
to visit with the biggest "Get Better Soon" card
I have ever seen.

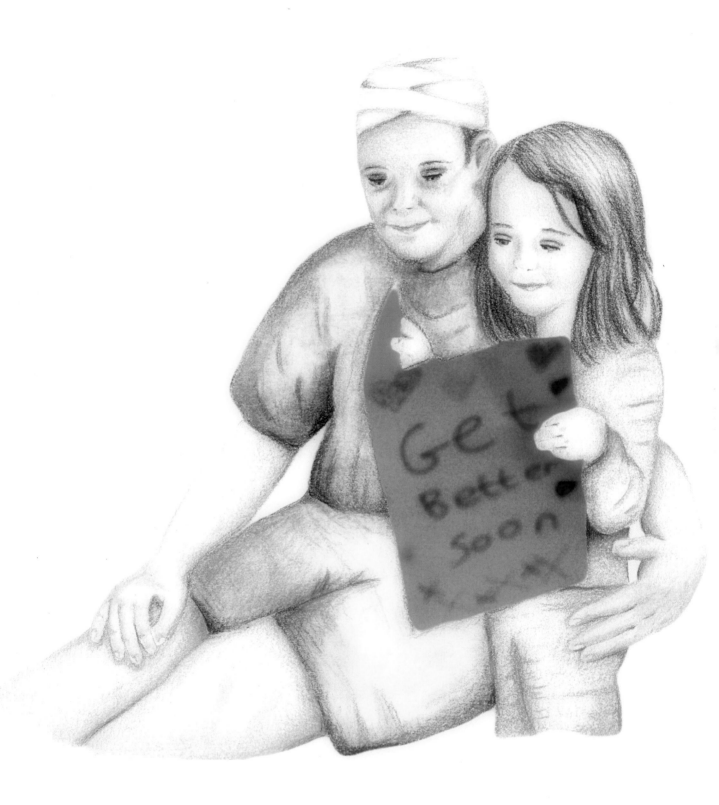

The card put a big smile on her dad's face, which made
Lilly smile too.

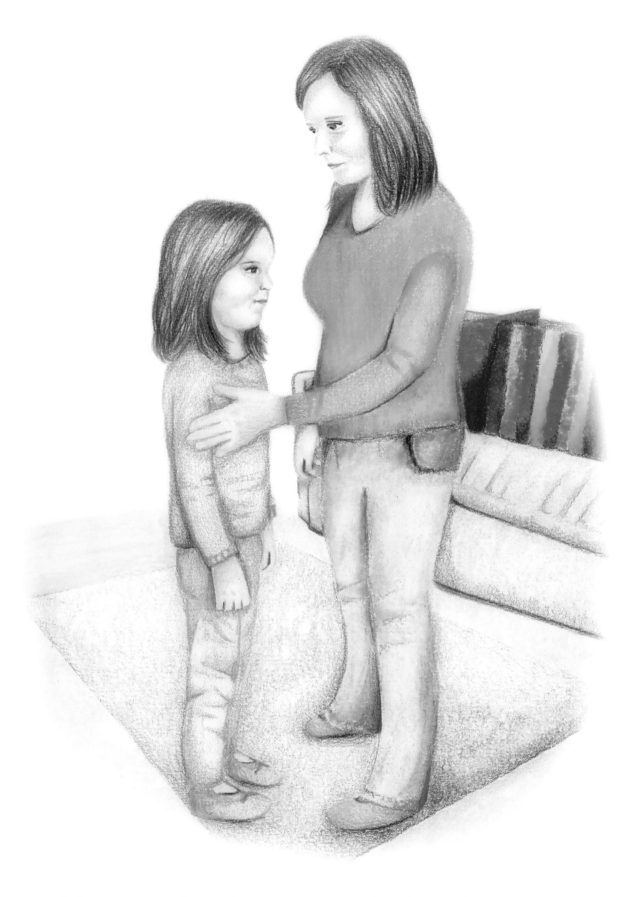

After some days in hospital, Lilly's dad went home to rest for a while.

But Lilly told her mum that she still felt sad.

"I'm happy daddy's home again but he's different now. I want my old daddy back," she whispered.

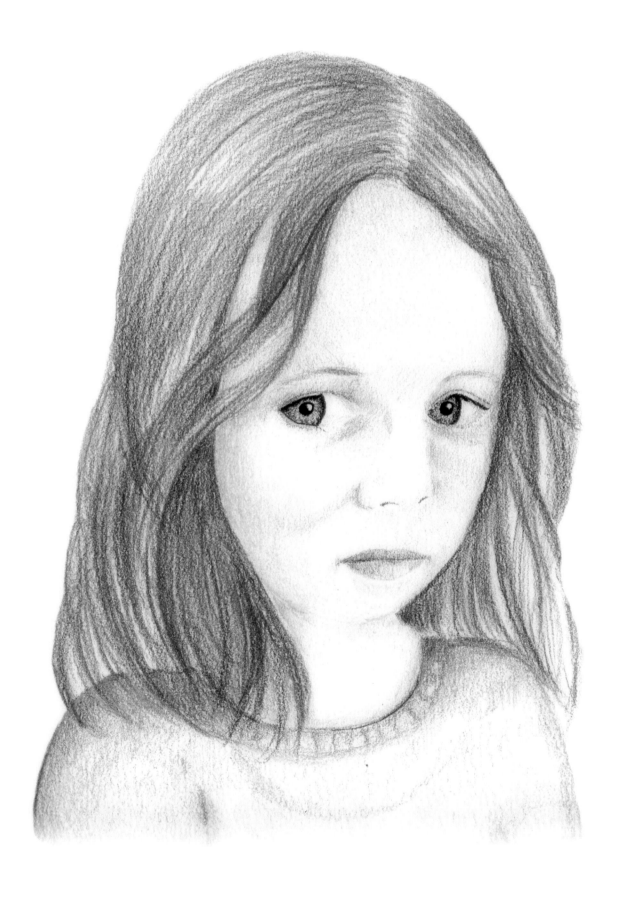

Lilly's mum explained that her dad was tired and weak because his body was fighting cancer.

"He may be forgetful at times and get a little confused," she said, "but there is one special thing that will always stay the same. Your daddy will always love you and that will never change."

As Lilly cried, her mum cuddled her closely and said it was ok to cry because it was ok to be sad.

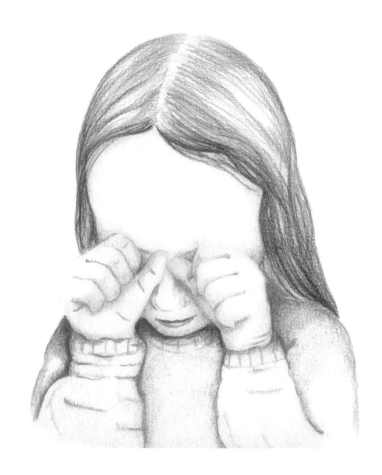

"It's ok to be angry too," she whispered, "because we both love daddy."

And she told Lilly that talking to each other would help because she wasn't on her own.

Lilly already felt much better.

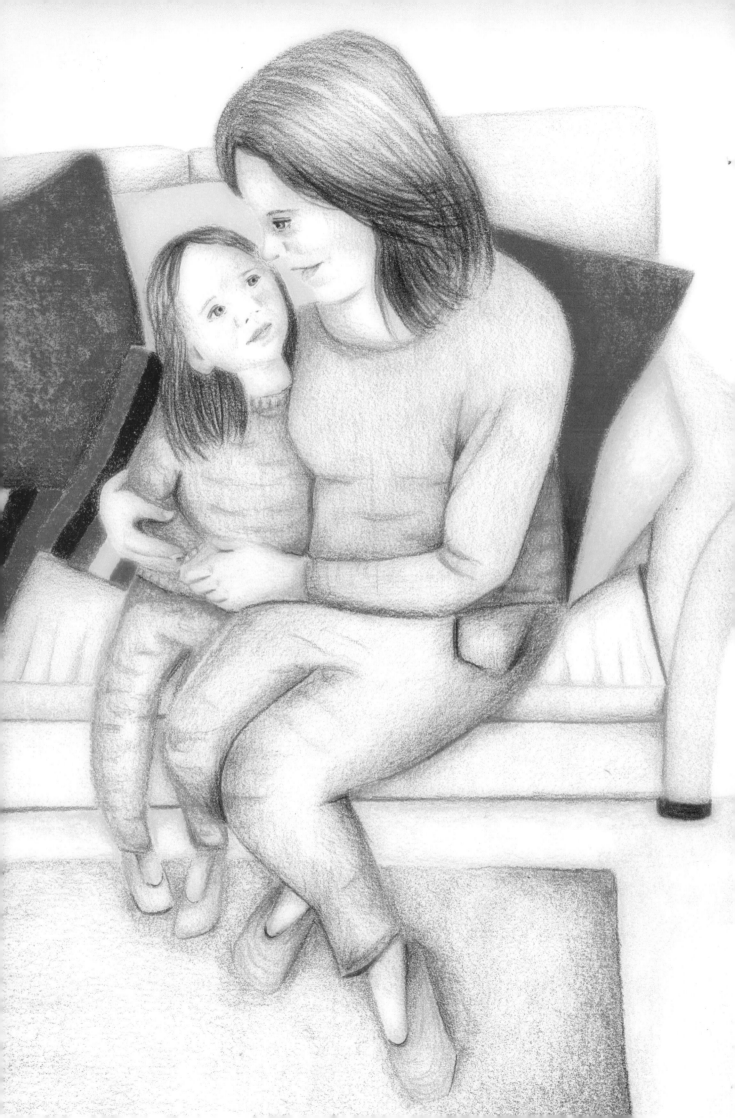

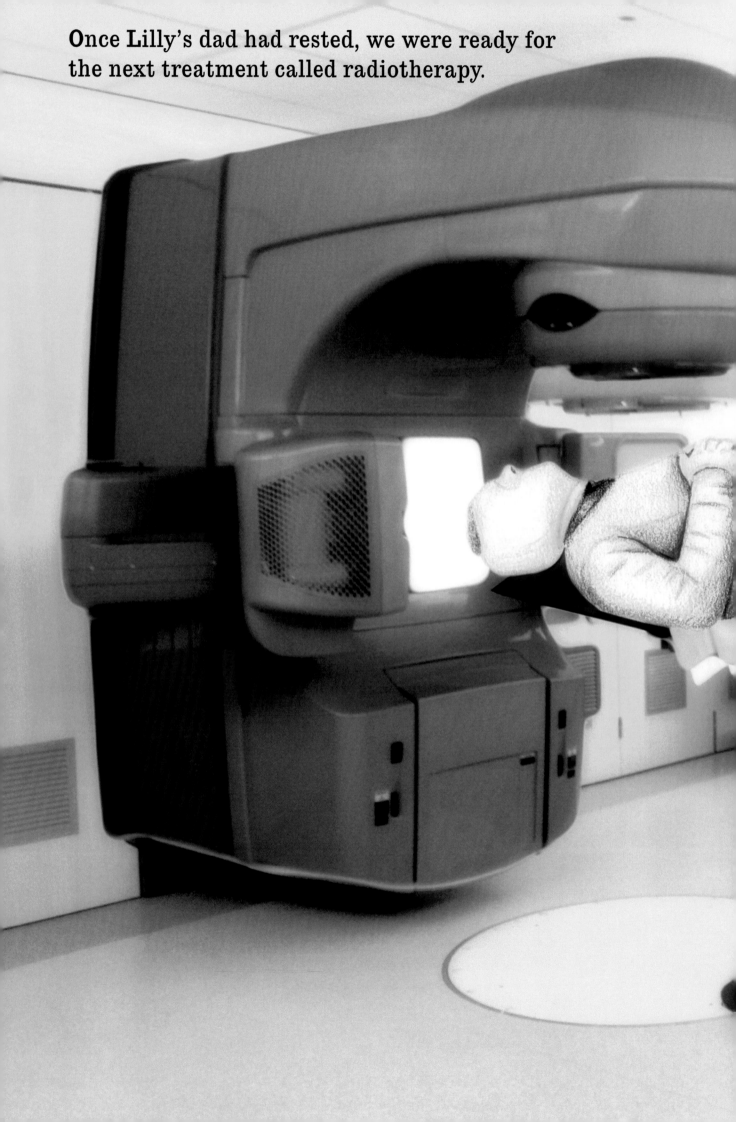

Once Lilly's dad had rested, we were ready for the next treatment called radiotherapy.

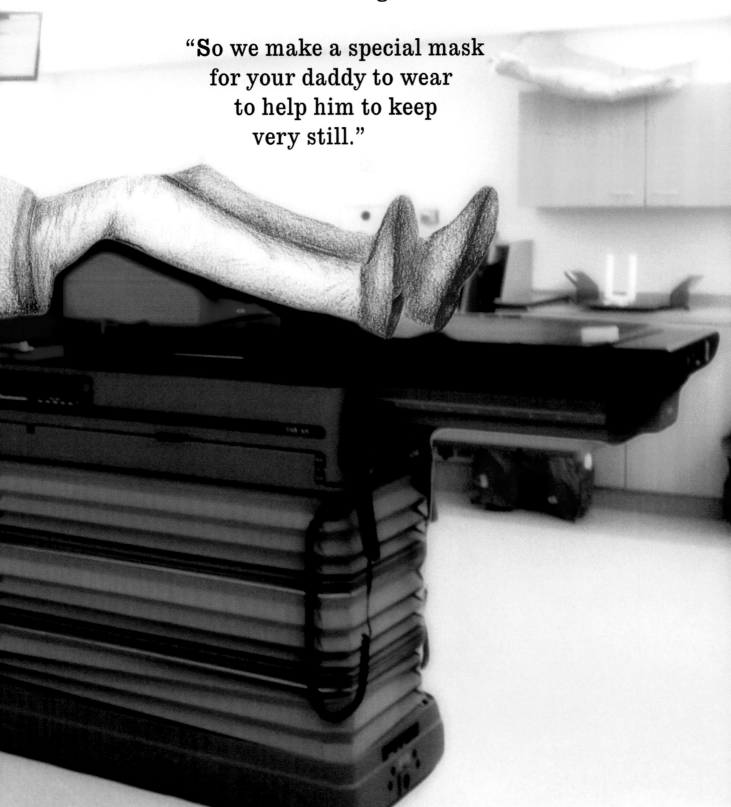

"Radiotherapy is like another scan," I explained, "to try to get rid of any sick cells left behind."

"Your daddy will lie down under a radiotherapy machine which will give him the medicine through invisible rays like sun rays."

"We have to make sure that the rays only hit the sick cells not the good ones."

"So we make a special mask for your daddy to wear to help him to keep very still."

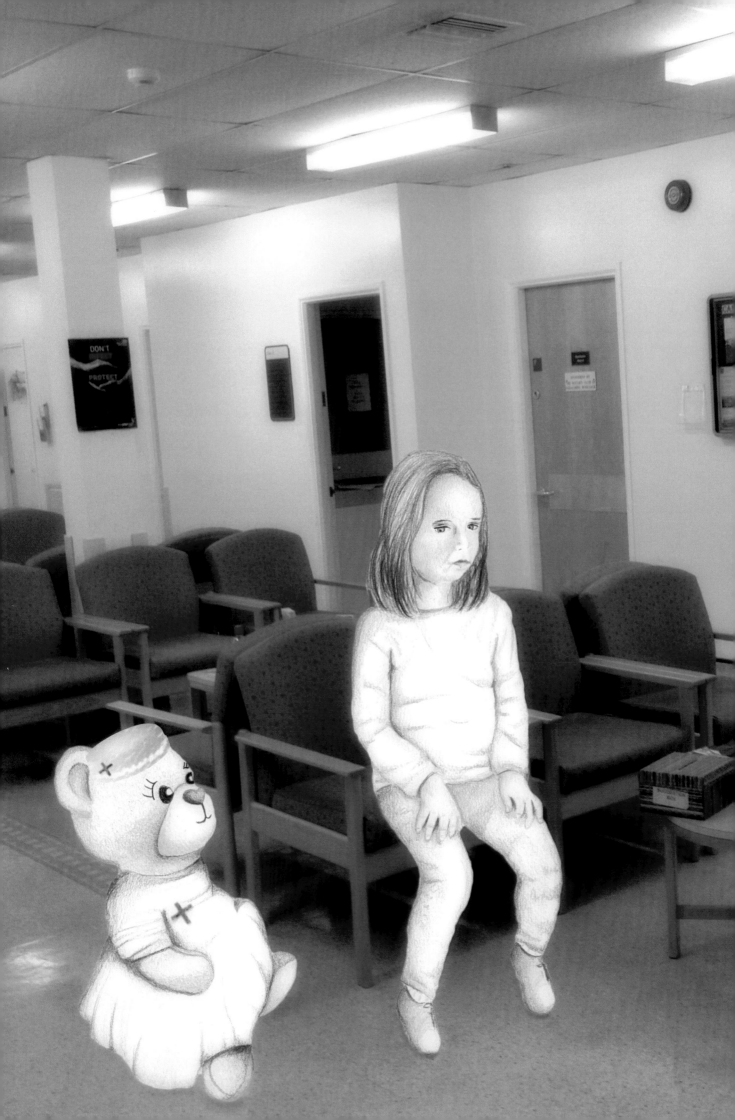

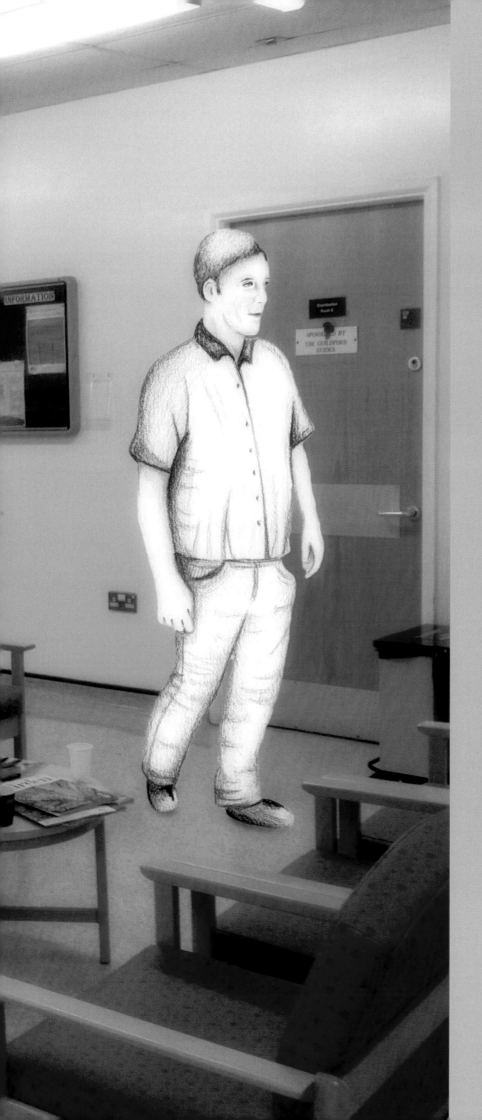

Lilly's dad came to visit us every day for his radiotherapy sessions.

The sessions didn't hurt but made him feel tired.

"Don't worry," I told Lilly, "he's tired because the medicine is working hard to try to get rid of the sick cells. The tiredness will get better after the treatment has finished."

At the same time as radiotherapy, Lilly's dad had the third type of treatment.

This was a medicine called chemotherapy to help get rid of the sick cells.

"The sick cells multiply too quickly," I explained, "so that one cell becomes two cells and then two cells become three cells and so on."

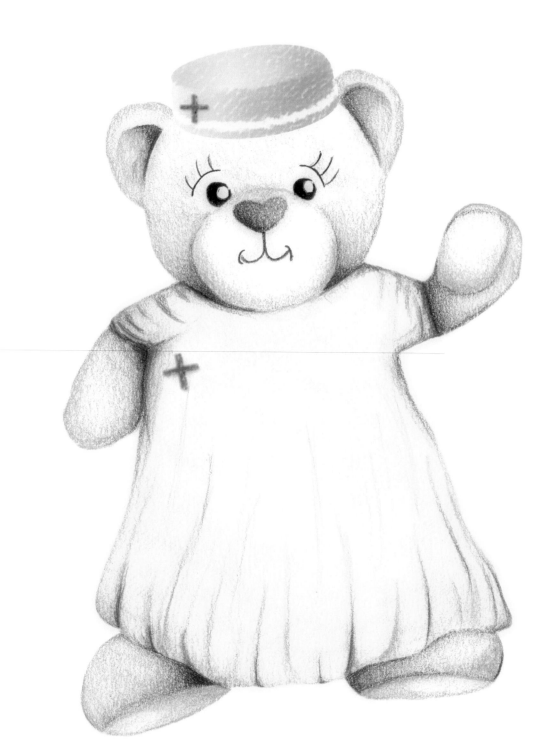

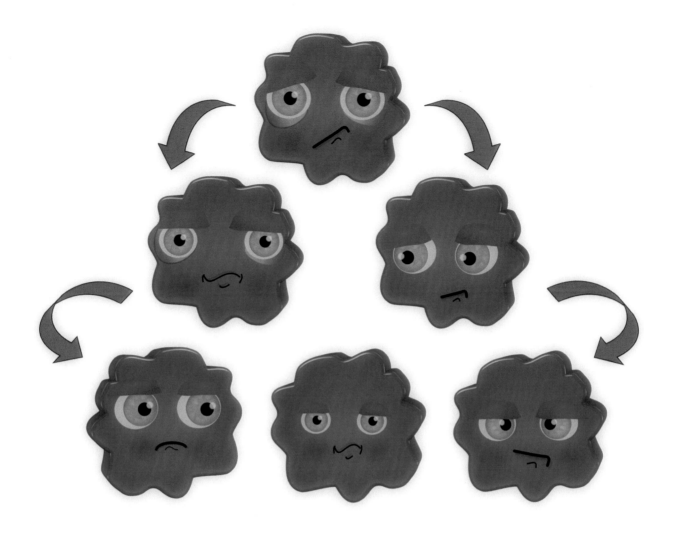

"The chemotherapy gets rid of these cells. The trouble is chemotherapy also gets rid of healthy cells that are meant to multiply quickly, like the cells that make your hair grow and white blood cells that help your body fight bugs like colds."

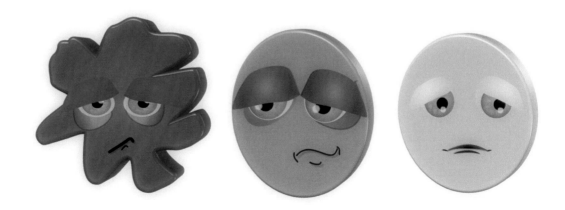

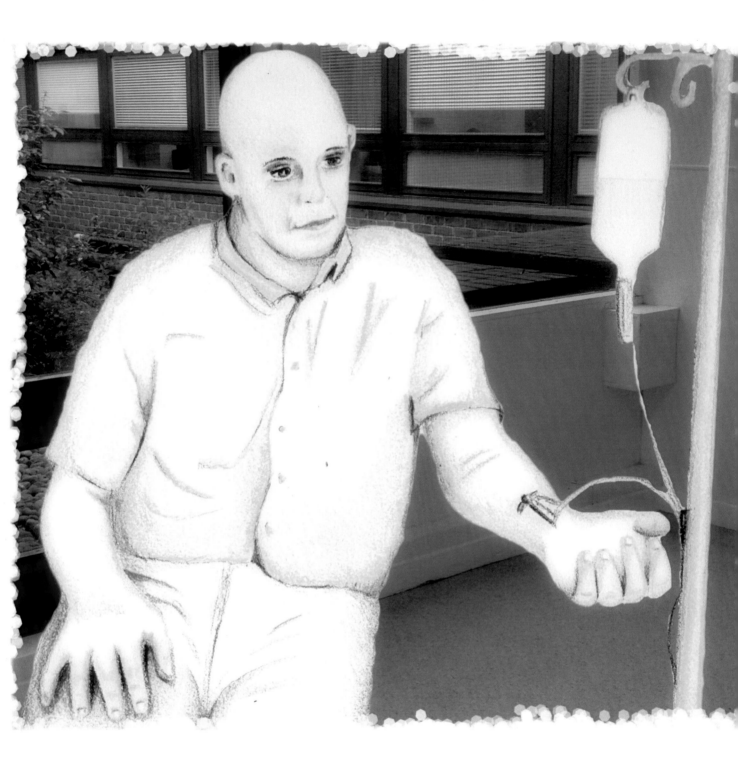

When Lilly's dad had a high temperature he had to stay in hospital so we could give him some special medicine. He had a room on his own to stop him catching any more bugs.

The chemotherapy also made him feel very ill but that was because it was helping his body to get rid of the sick cells.

His hair started to fall out too, which showed that the radiotherapy and chemotherapy were doing their job.

"He didn't have much hair in the first place!"
laughed Lilly.

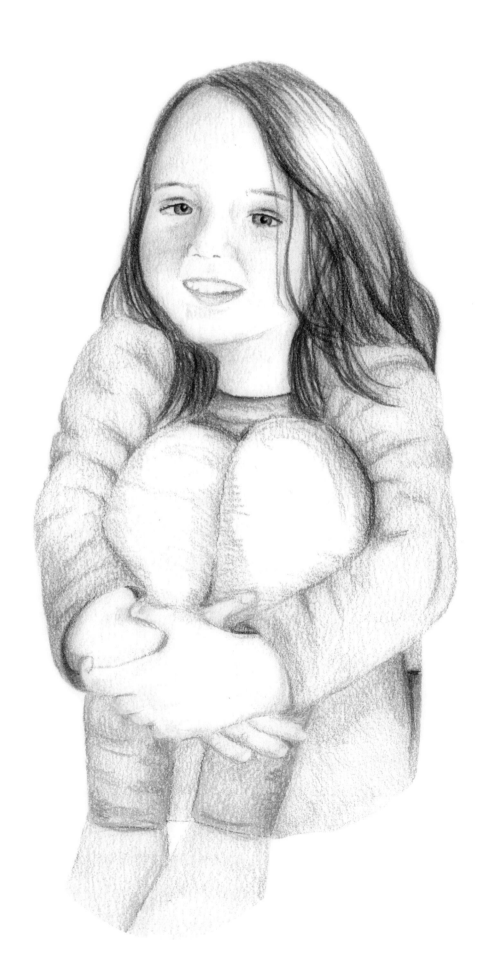

Lilly's dad has now started to feel a little better.

Now that he has had the three treatments, he can stay at home with Lilly and her mum and enjoy every moment together.

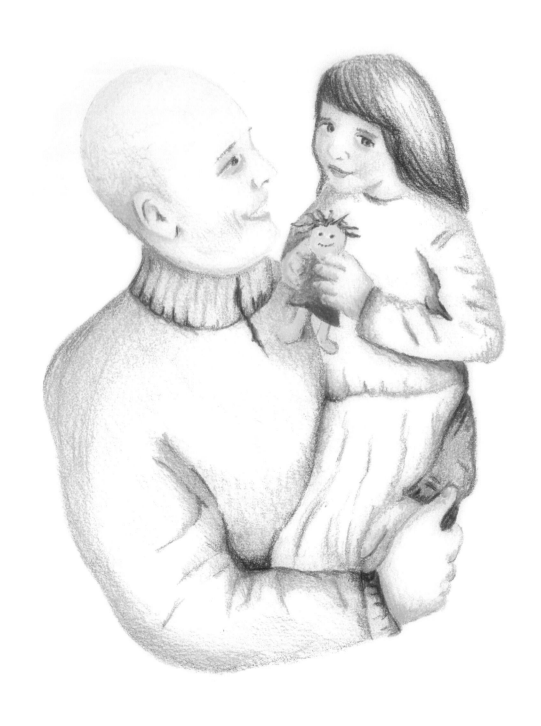

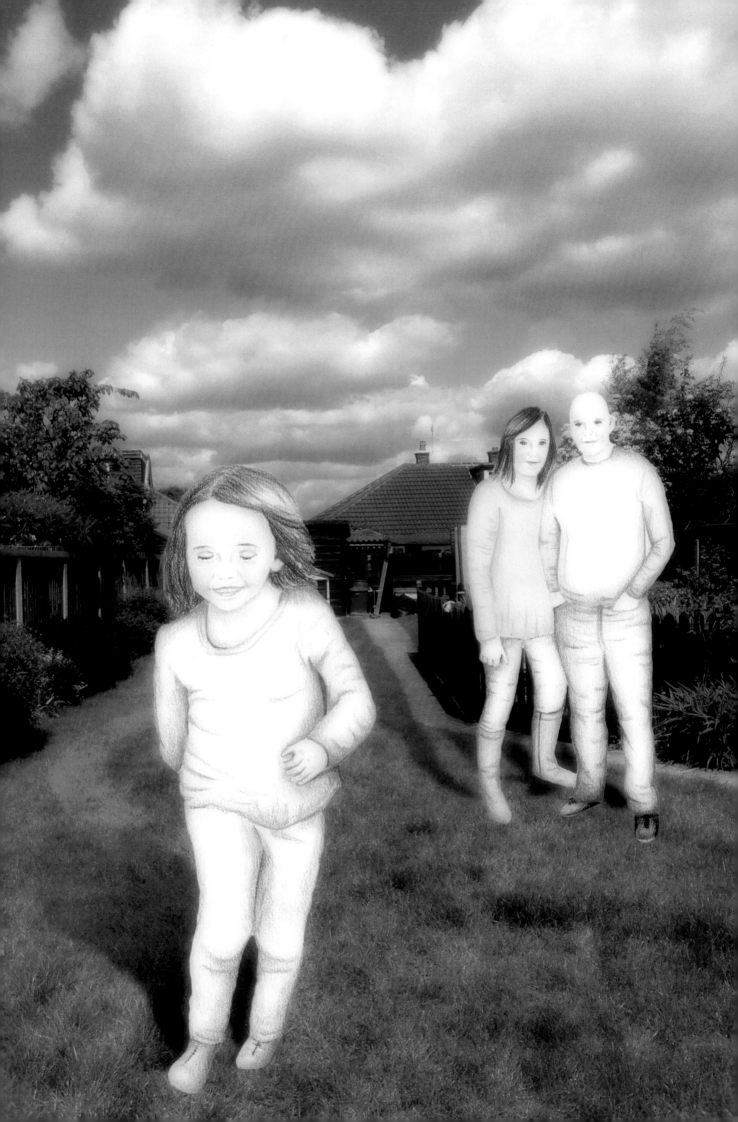

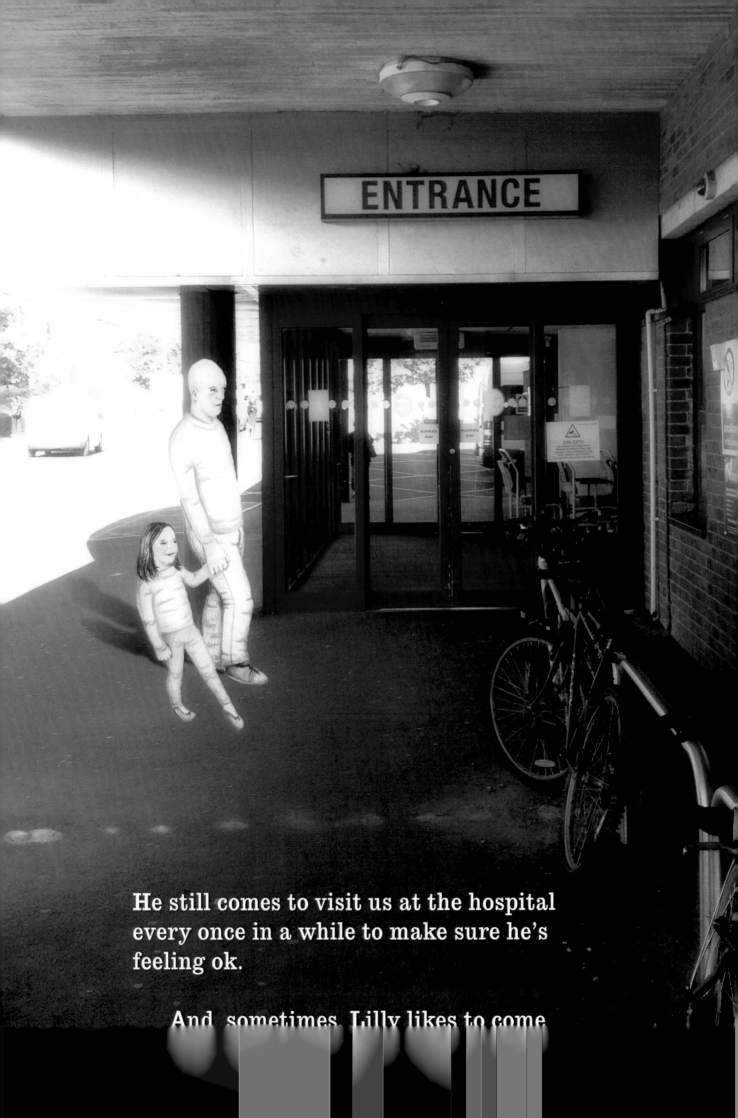

He still comes to visit us at the hospital
every once in a while to make sure he's
feeling ok.

And, sometimes, Lilly likes to come

After lots of practice at home,
Lilly gives the best bear hugs a ted could ever want.

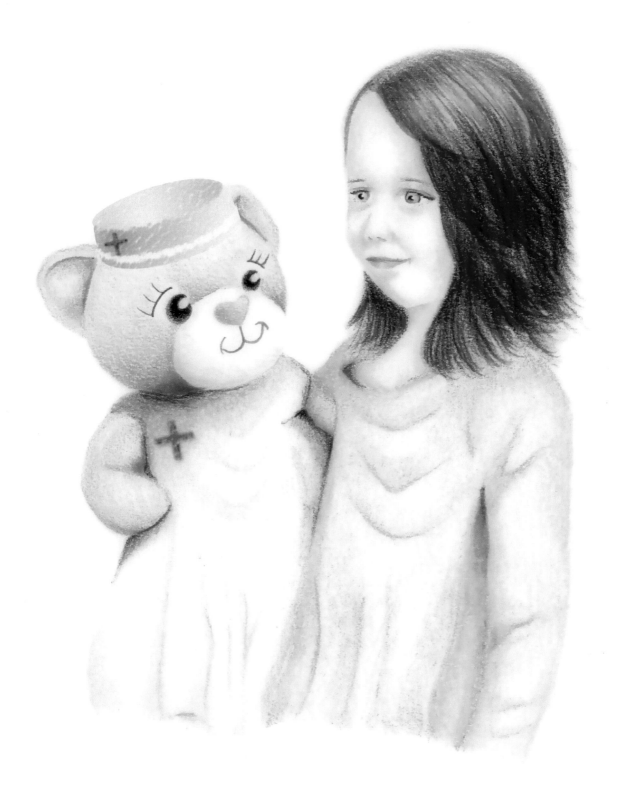

And her dad often tells me that,
whatever lies ahead,
those special hugs are the best medicine
he could wish for.

Glossary

Benign – **A** tumour that is not cancer.

Biopsy – **A** test to collect a sample of cells and look at it under a microscope to help make a diagnosis.

Blood test – **A** sample of blood that is taken from a vein and looked at in a laboratory.

Brain surgery – **An** operation performed by a brain surgeon to remove some of the brain tumour.

Cancer – **A** sickness caused by cells multiplying too quickly.

Cells – **The** building blocks of life. Human beings are made up of trillions of cells that help our bodies to work properly.

Chemotherapy – **Special** medicines used to treat cancer. They can be given as a tablet or by Intravenous Therapy (IV).

CT brain scan – **A** picture of the brain.

Diagnosis – **The** identification of an illness.

Epilepsy – **A** disorder that causes people to have seizures.

Infection – **A** germ inside someone's body which often causes a high temperature and makes the person feel unwell. The doctor may prescribe antibiotics to get rid of the germ.

Intravenous Therapy (IV) – **A** bag of liquid or medicines given into the vein.

Malignant – **A** tumour that is cancer.

MRI brain scan – **A** detailed picture of the brain.

Neuro-Oncology Clinical Nurse Specialist – **A** nurse who looks after people affected by brain tumours.

Occupational Therapist – **A** person who can help patients who have trouble doing everyday activities. They can suggest exercises, provide special equipment, and teach new ways to do things.

Oncologist – **A** doctor who treats people with cancer.

Oncology clinic – **A** place where people with cancer are seen by the doctor and nurse.

Patient – **A** person who is being looked after by a doctor or nurse.

Physiotherapist – **A** person who helps patients with their strength, balance and walking.

Radiotherapy – **A** special cancer treatment using x-rays. The x-rays are directed at cancer cells to try to stop them growing.

Radiotherapy Radiographer – **A** specially trained person who gives the x-ray treatment.

Seizure – When your body shakes or moves without control. Some people who have a brain tumour have seizures.

Scan – **A** picture of a part of your body. There are lots of different types of scans that a patient can have.

Speech and language therapist – **A** person who helps patients with their speech and communication.

Steroids – Special medicines to help reduce the swelling around the brain tumour.

Tests – **A** way to try to find out why someone is ill. For example, this could be a blood test or a scan.

Treatment – Medical care to help someone when they are ill. For example, antibiotics for an infection.

Tumour – **A** growth in the body which can be benign (not cancer) or malignant (cancer).

Side Effects of Treatment

Many of the treatments for brain tumours can cause side effects. But it is important to remember that treatment is there to help and is doing a lot of good.

Radiotherapy is a special cancer treatment using x-rays.
The x-rays are directed at brain cancer cells to try to stop them growing.

Side effects may include:

- Hair loss. The hair should grow back a few months after treatment.
- Sore/ red skin (like sun burn).
- Tiredness: both during the radiotherapy and for a while afterwards.
- Difficulty in remembering some things.
- Headaches and feeling sick.
- The side effects from the brain tumour may get worse during the treatment.

Chemotherapy is a special medicine used to treat cancer. It can be given as a tablet or into a vein (intravenous therapy).

The main side effect is that it can reduce the number of blood cells in the body:

- White blood cells fight infection. If the patient gets a sore throat or fever or catches a cold, they must go straight to hospital. They may need antibiotics.
- Red blood cells carry oxygen around the body. Low levels may make the patient feel tired and dizzy.
- Platelets help stop bleeding. Low levels may make the patient bruise easily or have nosebleeds and bleeding gums.
- A blood test is done before chemotherapy to check blood levels.

Steroids are a medicine to reduce the swelling around the brain tumour.

Side effects may include:

- Feeling more hungry and craving sugary foods like sweets or cakes.
- Difficulty sleeping.
- Swollen ankles and feet.
- Weaker arm or leg muscles.
- Increased blood sugar levels. The nurse will do a finger prick test to check this.

Questions you may have when a family member has a malignant (cancerous) brain tumour.

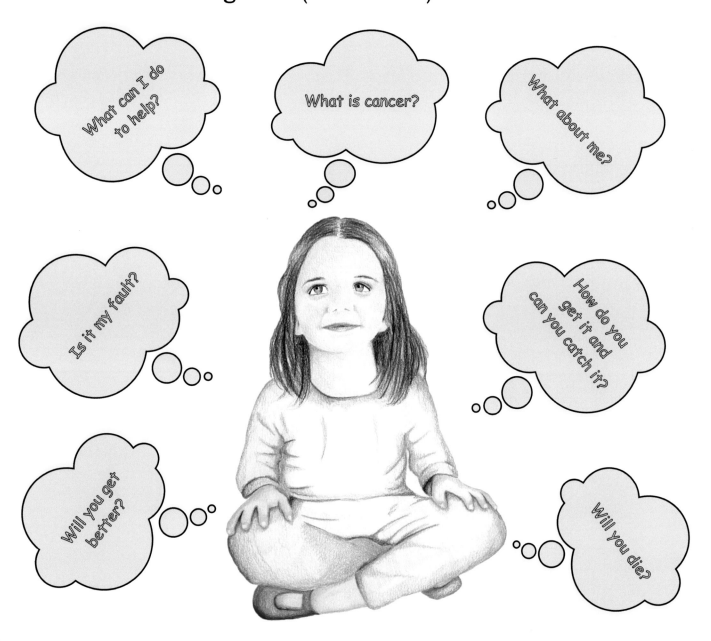

- **Cancer is a sickness caused by cells growing when they shouldn't.**

- **You can't catch cancer and we don't always know why people get cancer.**

- **It is nobody's fault; sometimes cells just get sick.**

- **Some people who have cancer do die and some people get better.**

- **With the help of the doctors and nurses, everything that can be done to treat the cancer is being done.**

- **The best thing you can do to help is to give your parents a big cuddle and lots of love.**

Thoughts and Feelings

You can use this page to draw a picture of your experiences
or to jot down your thoughts and feelings.